Veterinary
Aromatherapy

BY THE SAME AUTHOR

Aromathérapie, santé et bien être par les huiles essentielles, Albin Michel, Paris, 1993.

Aromatherapy, how to cure with essential oils, éditions de la chevêche, graveson, 1993.

Aromathérapie esthétique, des huiles essentielles pour votre beauté, éditions de la chevêche, graveson, 1992. Sold in aid of the "green seed exploration" foundation, Save the Planet.

Aromathérapie culinaire, l'alimentation "gagneur", des huiles essentielles dans votre assiette, éditions de la chevêche, graveson, 1991.

Aromathérapie 2, des huiles essentielles pour votre santé, éditions de la chevêche, graveson, 1987.

Aromatherapy from Provence, The C.W. Daniel Company, Saffron Walden, England, 1993.

IN PREPARATION

To be published by éditions de la chevêche, graveson:

100 remèdes d'urgence de médecine holistique et aromatique: mémento pour la santé au quotidien, April 1994.

La cuisine aromatique en Provence/Aromatic cooking in Provence (bilingual edition), January 1995.

Le livre du "musée des arômes et du parfum" de graveson en provence, Spring 1994.

Aromatherapie et hydrosolthérapie pour les enfants et la femme encente éditions de la chevêche, graveson, September 1994.

NELLY GROSJEAN

Veterinary Aromatherapy

*Natural remedies for cats, dogs, horses and birds,
and for the rearing of calves, cows, pigs, goats,
sheep, chicks, chickens, ducks and geese*

Translated from the French
by Joanne Robinson in association
with First Edition Translations Ltd, Cambridge

Index compiled by Lyn Greenwood

SAFFRON WALDEN
THE C.W. DANIEL COMPANY LIMITED

First published in France in 1993 by éditions la chevêche
under the title aromathérapie vétérinaire

This edited and revised English-language edition
first published in Great Britain in 1994
by The C.W. Daniel Company Limited
1 Church Path, Saffron Walden
Essex, CB10 1JP, England

ISBN 0 85207 274 0

Out of respect for the forests this book has been printed on
part re-cycled paper.

Design and Typesetting by Yew Design
Production in association with
Book Production Consultants Plc, Cambridge
Printed in England by St Edmundsbury Press,
Bury St Edmunds, Suffolk.

Contents

Preface

In conventional medicine, there is a strong tendency to forget that by suppressing pain and inflammation, we delay or prevent healing. The pain and inflammation is very much a part of the healing process and the desire at all costs to relieve an animal's suffering or "suppress" the disease only has the effect, in the long term, of delaying recovery.

Every individual will develop their own symptoms which are linked more to their own genetic make-up than to an actual cause. Most of the time, problems arise from a diet or lifestyle which does not meet the actual needs of the animal.

That is why prevention is always better than cure, and this principle is the common denominator amongst all natural therapies.

The abundant good advice and sensible aromatherapy remedies provided in this book will allow you, from now on, to practise natural medicine, in accordance with the laws of nature, on all domestic animals, farm-reared animals, and animals in training or racing environments, and I am very pleased to be able to congratulate the author on her achievement.

DR JACQUES LEGUERN
Natural therapy veterinarian

Foreword

Since the publication of my first four books on aromatherapy, I have been asked many times about its application for animals. Can we use essential oils to care for cats, dogs and horses, what doses should be given, how do the essential oils actually work, has aromatherapy been shown to be effective in the veterinary field? In this book you will find the answers to the most important questions that you ask yourself in trying to maintain in good health the animals that you have around you.

We know that aromatherapy is the use of essential aromatic oils (EOs) to prevent and cure disease. It is in fact one of the most important techniques used in complementary or natural medicine - also known as holistic or alternative medicine. Natural medicine is often thought of as "gentle", but that would not really be an appropriate term here, as essential oils are in actual fact small "showers of energy", bringing immediate and lasting benefits, as long as they are used advisedly. Essential oil and hydrolat (floral water) or hydrosol (hyd.) are both products of the distillation of an aromatic plant, distilled by a slow process of water vaporisation. The essential oils used therapeutically must be of excellent quality and come from healthy plants, either wild or grown organically, and must not be mixed with any synthetic chemical products.

Whenever essential oils are used, either according to the "recipes" in this book, or under the direction of a holistic veterinary surgeon, the instructions given should be followed very carefully. These days, most vets who are open to aromatherapy also practise homoeopathy and osteopathy, and take into account the "emotional relationship" between the animal and its owner. Furthermore, aromatherapy works extremely well in conjunction with homoeopathy.

On the subject of aromatherapy, we should remember that before they were commonly used to prevent and treat ailments in humans, essential oils first appeared on the scene as a result of the excellent work and research of Professors Gattefossé (at the beginning of the 20th century) and Sévelinge (around 50 years ago), who used them to treat animals. Many earlier works exist, including one from the 18th century listing veterinary remedies based on plant extracts, used notably by the "Ecole de Cavalerie".

Cats, dogs, horses and farm-reared animals of all kinds can benefit from the remarkable properties of aromatic essential oils. Their effects are immediate and the results long-lasting. They are a perfect complement to good animal husbandry. With their ability to fight infection and to act as an antiseptic amongst their principal properties, essential oils can be used as a preventative and as a curative treatment for both the usual traditional diseases and those specific to the animal. Just as for humans, using essential oils for animals is a speedy and effective method in helping to provide a balanced lifestyle, a healthy and appropriate diet, and of course, the essential basic conditions of freedom and cleanliness.

All animals require a diet particular to their morphology and organic functions. The bird has a beak designed to eat seeds. The lion has kidneys that eliminate, amongst other things, nitrogenous waste generated from the digestion of animal proteins. Horses feed on grains and vegetable products and, finally, fish can be herbivores or carnivores. As far as the more familiar animals are concerned, we will stress the need for a healthy, essentially raw - although sometimes, cereals and vegetables need to be cooked (wild animals cannot cook their own meals!) - and natural diet, to which should be added food supplements to counteract a largely sedentary way of life, and essential oils to increase resistance to disease.

For animals raised in a battery or other intensive system, essential oils should only be used in diffusion, either by means of aerosols, aroma diffusers or through the ventilation, heating or air-conditioning system.

Although this book tackles the most important straightforward health problems of our animal friends, it should not be considered a substitute for diagnosis and treatment by your own vet. You will find instructions for use, dosage, and appropriate length of treatment and prevention in the individual chapters on cats, dogs, horses, birds, and rearing our "two-footed" and "four-footed" friends. At the front of this book, you will find all the "key" aromatic blends, as well as the aromatic veterinary medicines. Also at the beginning of the book is a summary of the principal ailments and treatments and, at the end, a clear index providing rapid access to the information sought.

All essential oils have powerful antiseptic, detoxifying and revitalising properties. For this reason, they increase resistance to disease, strengthen the immune system and prevent infection and infectiousness. For preventative or curative purposes, they can be taken in three different ways: by diffusion into the air (natural essential oil), as a massage (natural and/or diluted essential oil), or by internal absorption (natural or, preferably, diluted essential oil). But, before proceeding any further, let us remind ourselves of the common properties and specific qualities of aromatic essential oils.

Qualities of essential oils

Most aromatherapy "recipes" are the product of simple common sense combined with a precise knowledge of how to use aromatic essential oils. For animals, just as for humans, it is preferable to use good quality oils that have not been adulterated or "chemically" treated. Certainly, they must always be kept in tinted glass containers, and away from heat and light. The label should show the precise name of the plant; it is usual, too, to know where it was distilled, the latin name and the part of the plant which was distilled (bark or peel, leaf, whole plant, berry or root). The manufacturer is obliged to provide this information if you request it.

The effects and benefits of the essential oils that we will cover refer only to those essential oils obtained by distillation through water vaporisation or expressed by mechanical means from plants or fruits that have not been additionally heated. It goes without saying that these high quality essential oils have been neither diluted nor reconstituted synthetically in any way.

It is valuable to know the origin of the distilled plant since it is this, together with its "vintage", that gives the plant its properties. In fact, the relative proportion of constituents can vary quite considerably with the soil of origin.

The part of the plant that is distilled also provides important information about a plants properties; it is important to know whether it is the bark or the leaves as, for example, in cinnamon where the relative proportion of certain constituents varies greatly between the two.

Although less strictly defined, the organoleptic characteristics represent an important parameter in the demand for quality in essential oils. This also applies to:

- the colour on emergence from the still, although this changes with oxidation and ageing: a rich red savory becomes almost black; the indigo blue of wild camomile turns a brownish hue, etc.

- the smell and taste, although these can only be detected by an expert "nose".

- the opalescence, which is a sure indication that the oil is not genuine except in the case of the natural opalescence of *Litsea cubeba*, patchouli, amyris and sandalwood, created by iron in suspension. Lavender can have an opalescence in the final stage of distillation due to particles of water in suspension. This opalescence can be removed by filtering through sodium sulphate or, better still, by distilling dried or semi-dried plants.

Physical measurements complete the assessment of organoleptic characteristics: these are essentially optical rotation, density, the refractive index and solubility in ethyl alcohol.

Chemical analyses, to determine the presence of, for example, estersand acids, or amounts of terpenes, phenols and cineoles, are also part of the physical assessment.

Since the 19th century, the expanding perfume industry and refinements in chromatographic analysis have combined to produce new products for the manufacturing distillers.

To verify the quality of essential oils, there are currently three tests that can be run: bioelectronic analysis; chromatography - either gas or liquid chromatography, capillary or molecular chromatography (NMR), or thin layer chromatography; and finally, radiation detectors. Such analyses allow the detection of any adulteration, just as a good "nose" can be equally effective in a more empirical way.

Essential oils that come from plants grown organically (not treated with artificial fertilizer - labels such as *Nature et progrès*, *Demeter* or *Biodynamie*...) or essences from wild plants offer the best guarantee of quality. These should always be used in preference to others.

All essential oils are:
- antiseptic, antimicrobial, anti-infectious (the majority)
- detoxifying
- revitalising
- regulators of the nervous system and hormonal glands.

Note

The properties of an essential oil are not necessarily the same as those of the plant from which it is taken, whilst the plant itself does not necessarily possess the properties of its corresponding essential oil.

Essential oils or aromatic essences are not fatty oils and their constituents, being essentially volatile, therefore do not leave a stain on paper.

"Super-action" of essential oils

Being concentrates of general or specific active constituents, essential oils have a fast-acting therapeutic action. They are primarily laevorotatory, unlike synthetic chemical substances which are generally dextrorotatory.

Concentrates of plants in the form of juices, tinctures of fresh herbs or infusions are not as powerful as essential oils. Just as in homoeopathy, they can often be used to complete an essential oil treatment. As to their speed of action, three to six weeks (maximum three months) is generally sufficient to restore an imbalance in the system in conditions recently treated with essential oils.

Remarkable elective properties

This is a unique phenomenon in the area of natural therapy. An essential oil applied to a part of the body is drawn to that part of the body, organ or function which is deficient. This exceptional ability to be "magnetised" is a property exclusive to essential oils, and neither plants nor plant juices possess this ability.

Powerful action

Essential oils are not a panacea but, in 80% of cases, they bring about a recognised improvement with an increase in vital energy within the first five to ten days of treatment, the problem generally resolving itself finally within anything from three weeks to three months. In all cases, as no one therapy can be said to be the philosopher's stone, a well-planned aromatherapy treatment will be enhanced by a new, healthy lifestyle (diet, vertebral release, physical exercise and fresh air, attention to and consideration for the animal). Despite its extremely powerful action, aromatherapy is nevertheless subject to the great law of "gentle" medicines and is thus: "a global medicine encompassing all the natural therapies".

I particularly like the following recommendation to doctors by Dr J. Valnet, author of *Docteur nature* and *The Practice of Aromatherapy* (The C.W. Daniel Co Ltd, Saffron Walden, England): "Scientific discovery may still have a long way to go, but doctors can bide their time and draw inspiration from the empirical teachings of the past, caring for patients by using those treatments known to be effective, even if we don't yet understand the reasons why."

Note

Essential oil from Spanish wild marjoram origanum vulgare possesses:
- an anticolibacillus activity of the first order according to the aromatogram, stronger than thyme, cinnamon, savory, clove, pine or cajeput
- an anti-amoebic action of the first order
- an anti-infectious action of the first order against:
  - *Staphylococcus aureus*
  - *β-haemolytic streptococcus Group A*
  - *pneumococcus*
  - *Candida albicans*
  - *enterococcus and Streptococcus faecalis.*

According to the aromatogram results, in every case this proves to be the essential oil with the most powerful antiseptic properties!

Essential oil of savory acts on microbial germs at a concentration twenty times less than that of the other labiates used in pharmacology (lavender, rosemary, sage) and at a concentration two to three times less than that of thyme.

"Essential oil of lemon neutralises the typhoid bacillus - Eberth -, *Staphylococcus aureus*, the diphtheria bacillus -

Loeffler - and the pneumococcus, in less than three hours"
(Dr J. Valnet).

Physico-chemical action

Astonishing results in all diseases where the blood pH is
alkaline, the Rh2 corresponds to an oxidising solution, and
resistance is low (research by L. C. Vincent).

Action on vital energy

The vibratory action of every essential oil stimulates by
induction the internal vibrations which characterise all the
cells in the living body, consisting of thousands of small
cellular motors. Aromatherapy ranks among the top
"elemental" medicines by virtue of the fact that it acts
directly by increasing the vital force, thereby strengthening
the natural immune system and promoting self-healing. In
most animals, a dose of magnesium chloride will complete
this elemental treatment (20 g per litre of water, 3 to 10
times a day per 20 kg of body weight for a period of 10
days, 3 to 4 times per year).

Principal ailments in animals and their treatment

In this table, the indications for use of essential oils are self-explanatory, and are given mainly in cases where there is no explanation on a separate reference page (example: for thrush, bites and stings ... external use; for urinary calculus ... internal use).

You will find *Practical advice* on pages 17 to 18.

We refer throughout to essential oils, unless we are referring to infusion, juices or hydrosols*, in which case these are specified each time.

* hydrosol is the special name given to the first 20 litres of hydrolat (floral water) distilled from an organically grown aromatic plant at source. You may well come across hydrolat which has been produced synthetically, not naturally. Hydrosol is always natural and of organic quality.

abscesses	*dog p 54; cat p 27; horse p 72*
abraded pads	*see p 28 or 55*
anaemia	*cat p 24; dog p 50*
anxiety, distress	*basil + sweet marjoram*
asthma	*hyssop and see respiratory properties p 13*
bites	*lavender + clay*
bronchitis	*see respiratory properties p 13*
burns	*key blend B*
calculi (urinary)	*juniper or sandalwood*
calculi (vesicular)	*juniper or rosemary*

cholera	*mint, wild marjoram, thyme*
cirrhosis	*wild marjoram, rosemary*
colic	*cinnamon, caraway*
common cold	*see respiratory properties p 13*
coryza	*cat p 31; dog see respiratory properties p 13*
conjunctivitis	*hydrosol of cornflower + lemon juice*
constipation	*see diet pp 21, 38 or 69*
coughs	*see respiratory properties p 13 + lavender or orange; cat p 30; horse p 74*
cracked skin (mammals)	*key blend B*
cuts	*key blend A*
cyst	*clay*
dentition (tartar)	*see dog p 11*
depression	*basil + sweet marjoram*
dermatoses	*key blend A + B + magnesium chloride; dog p 60; horse p 81*
diabetes	*eucalyptus + juniper + lemon*
diarrhoea	*cinnamon*
digestion	*mint or caraway*
dyspepsia	*see digestion*
eczema	*see dermatoses*
emphysema	*see respiratory properties p 13; cat p 30*
excitement	*see sedatives p 14*
fatigue	*rosemary + coriander; dog p 49*

fetid breath	*mint, nutmeg; dog p 64*
fever	*diet + magnesium chloride + lemon and sage*
fistula	*see abscess*
flatulence	*see digestive properties p 13*
fleas	*terebinth + olive oil or massage using essential oil of mint or put mint leaves in bedding or lemongrass essential oil; dog p 62; cat p 29*
foreign bodies	*clay*
fractures	*clay; dog p 56; cat p 32*
gastroenteritis	*diet + consult vet*
gingivitis	*clay + key blend C*
giving birth	*verbena infusion; see p 41 (dog) and p 22 (cat)*
haemorrhaging (light)	*key blend A*
haemorrhaging (serious)	*consult vet*
harvest mite	*terebinth or lemongrass, rose geranium, cinnamon, clove*
heart, cardiopathy	*mint*
heatstroke	*mint*
hepatitis	*see liver*
indigestion	*diet + hydrosol of rosemary + caraway essential oil*
insomnia	*lavender, sweet marjoram*

intoxication

- from medication   *mint*

- chemical   *consult vet (cat p 25; dog p 51)*

liver   *rosemary, mint*

lumbago   *rosemary + clay*

mange   *clove, pine or terebinth or juniper or*
                     lemon + lavender + wild marjoram

nervous

depression   *basil + sweet marjoram*

nervousness   *lavender, sweet marjoram, neroli*

obesity   *dog: reduce rations by half + lemon +*
                     juniper

odours   *cat p 33*

otitis   *lemon juice or warm olive oil in the ear*

over-exertion   *horse p 79*

pain

- articular   *see analgesics p 13 and horse p 77*

- muscular   *horse p 76*

paralysis   *osteopathy or acupuncture + clay +*
                     reduce protein intake + purge; dog p 59

parasites   *see harvest mites, fleas and ticks*

poisoning   *veterinary; dog p 51; cat p 25*

phlegmon   *see abscess*

pneumonia   *see respiratory properties p 13*

pyroplasmosis   *consult vet*

quadrate muscle,

disease of   *consult vet*

rabies	consult vet + slaughter of infected animal
rheumatism	juniper + birch + terebinth + pine + rosemary + hydrosol of juniper or elder + roll animal in nettles + see p 57 for the dog and see antirheumatic properties
scratches	clay + key blend A
skin	horse p 80; dog pp 60
skin irritation	horse p 80
snake bites	clay + mint
sores	key blends A + B + clay
sprains	clay
spikelets, spicules	see abraded pads
staphylococci	wild marjoram, cinnamon, thyme, mint + diffusion of key blend C
stiffness/aches and pains	horse pp 76 and 77
stings	lavender, or rub in three-herb combination (old Provencal remedy) using parsley, garlic and onion or crushed cabbage, leek or tomato
streptococci	see staphylococci above
stress	horse p 70; birds p 92
tartar	clay powder + lemon rubbed + scaling
tetanus	wild marjoram, cinnamon, mint, lemon

thorns, splinters	*see abraded pads*
thrush	*clove or lemon*
ticks	*terebinth + oil of St John's wort;*
	cat: vinegared water on fur
toxoplasmosis	*consult vet*
travel sickness	*basil 48 h before + bunch of parsley*
	underneath animal
tumours	*consult vet*
typhus	*cat (often fatal): diet + consult vet*
	see p 31
ulcers	*clay + key blend A*
vaginal	
discharge	*sage*
vaginitis	*clean with hydrosol of sage + essential*
	oil of lavender
worms	*see cat p 26; dog p 46 and horse p 73*
vomiting	*diet + mint or lavender or lemon juice*
	or hydrosol of tarragon
weight loss	*cat p 24; dog p 50*
wounds	*see key blends A and B*
the essential	
oils of the	
aromatogram	*wild marjoram, savory, cinnamon,*
	thyme, clove, cajeput, pine, lavender,
	mint.

Principal properties of essential oils (EOs)

analgesic	*lavender, marjoram, camomile*
"antibiotic"	*wild marjoram no. 1 in the aromatogram; savory, cinnamon, thyme, clove, mint*
antirheumatic	*juniper, birch, rosemary, pine, terebinth, sandalwood*
antiseptic	
• intestinal	*caraway, cinnamon*
• genito-urinary	*sandalwood, ylang-ylang, juniper*
• respiratory	*thyme, wild marjoram, cinnamon, eucalyptus*
antispasmodic	*camomile, tarragon*
antidepressant	*basil + sweet marjoram*
cicatrisant (promotes scar formation)	*lavender, rose geranium, rosemary + see key blends A and B*
digestive	*caraway, nutmeg, coriander, cumin, mint*
diuretic	*lemon, birch, juniper, sandalwood*
respiratory	*eucalyptus, pine, thyme, hyssop, terebinth, tea-tree; horse p 74; cats p 30; birds p 91; pigs, cattle p 94*
revitalising	*coriander, savory, cinnamon, rosemary, wild marjoram, ylang-ylang*

sedative	
• pain relief	*see analgesics*
• sleep	*lavender, sweet marjoram, neroli*
• relaxation	*lavender, sweet marjoram, camomile*
slimming	*lemon, juniper, rose geranium, birch*

Aromatic veterinary medicines

Essential oil of terebinth: cleansing, improves fur or coat (dog, horse)

Essential oil of eucalyptus: respiratory

Essential oil of lavender: sedative, aseptic, cicatrisant

Essential oil of wild marjoram: the most "antibiotic" of the essential oils

Essential oil of cinnamon: arrests diarrhoea

Essential oil of juniper: drains malfunctioning kidneys

Essential oil of mint: digestive, aseptic

Clay for poultices (instructions for use pp 18 and 56)

Oil of St John's wort is particularly good for healing scar tissue, improves blood circulation in general and has the ability to reconstitute intervertebral cartilage (Docteur Breuss, 1920, Federal Republic of Germany). In addition, it is an ideal active support medium for the majority of essential oils.

Magnesium chloride: strengthens natural resistance

Hydrosol of cedar: apply to horse's or dog's coat, improves appearance and promotes regrowth (does the same for our hair too!)

"Key" aromatic blends

A. An all-round blend for healing scar tissue and promoting relaxation

oil of St John's wort	*60 ml*
EO of lavender or lavandin	*15 ml*

B. A blend that heals scars and regenerates damaged tissue (loss of fur, cutaneous lesions, scar tissue from burns)

oil of St John's wort	*60 ml*
wheat germ oil	*30 ml*
EO of lavender or lavandin	*15 ml*
EO of rose geranium	*5 ml*
EO of rosemary	*5 ml*

C. Cleansing, aseptic blend

oil of St John's wort	*15 ml*
olive oil or alcohol	*90 ml*
EO of terebinth	*60 ml*
EO of lavender	*15 ml*

for use on sores, cuts, gashes; alternate with a clay poultice.

Note

Only essential oil of terebinth is effective in eliminating ticks and such like in dogs.

Only essential oil of lavender or of lavandin has both cleansing and antiseptic properties, as well as being calming and promoting healing of scar tissue and trauma sites (see *Aromatic veterinary medicines* on previous page).

Practical advice

There are three methods of absorbing essential oils: internally, by diffusion or by massage.
Essential oils in food and in water: for internal use
Hydrosols in water: for internal use
Essential oils in diffusion: for external use
Clay or cabbage poultices: for external use
Mixtures to promote healing of scar tissue, with antiseptic and cleansing properties, for external use: key aromatic blends

Essential oils in food

They can be mixed easily in food, just like seasoning.
Standard dose: 1 to 5 drops of essential oil 2 to 3 times a day depending on the animal and its weight.
Length of treatment during crisis periods is from 3 to 7 days.
In preventative or post-crisis period, one dose per day for 1 to 3 weeks.
During a period of fasting, essential oils can be added:
- to drinking water (despite being insoluble in water)
- to carrot juice (dog, cat, horse) with daily yeast.
- to water with daily yeast (concentrate of B group vitamins); cats, dogs and horses are fond of it.

Hydrosols in drinking water

In certain cases (birds, fowl and "two-footed" creatures, also cats) hydrosols (water from the first stage of distillation which still contains microparticles of essential oil in suspension) will be recommended (see *Table of principal ailments*). Hydrosol therapy is a type of "homoeopathic aromatherapy".
Standard dose: The standard dose of hydrosol for an animal of 50 kg is 3 to 4 tablespoons per litre of water. This should be increased or reduced according to weight. It should be remembered that frequent, low doses repeated during the course of the day will be more effective than one strong

dose once a day (see Plateau's effect in our book *Aromatherapy from Provence*, published by The C.W. Daniel Company, Saffron Walden, England, 1993).

Essential oils in diffusion

For all commercial breeding in stables, catteries and aviaries, the electric diffuser permits simple and easy dispersal of essential oils into the atmosphere. Respiratory and antiseptic essential oils can be diffused in this way. Essential oils used as a sedative or tonic are better administered by massage, as ointment or taken internally; essential oils to aid digestion, or for draining or revitalising, should be taken internally (via food).

The aroma diffuser should operate for between 1 to 2 hours per day, depending on circumstances (see indications for use in the relevant chapters).

Clay poultices

In a glass or earthenware bowl, cover the clay (powder or small pieces, either green, pink or white) with water. Allow the water to soak in. Stir with a wooden spoon (not plastic or metal) until mixture forms a thick paste.

Place gauze on the part to be treated (to avoid fur being pulled when poultice is dry).

Apply clay to a thickness of 1 to 2 centimetres.

Place a double thickness of paper tissue on the poultice and secure with a bandage.

Leave in place for 1 to 3 hours.

Remove with warm water and replace with a fresh poultice or alternate with an application of the appropriate aromatic blend.

Cabbage poultice

Can be used instead of clay if there is none available. Crush the large leaves and apply directly to the wound, injury or burn. Renew every 2 to 4 hours.

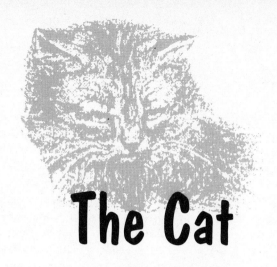

The Cat

I am a sociable creature

Golden rules to follow in order that I might love you for a long time

I am not a toy: I need affection, and sometimes I like to play if I am kitten or a young cat.

I like things to be kept clean if I live in a house or a flat, and I like to be told where to do my business.

I need food every day and, if I am a male cat, I also like hunting.

I like to go outside and run in the country, or at least in fresh air (even if it means being on a lead).

I don't like being left alone when you go away on holiday or for long weekends. Either take me with you or leave me with friends (or in a cattery).

Don't hit me unnecessarily: teach me the rules of your house, I will be able to understand them.

When I am ill, care for me and consider my lifestyle. There must be something lacking. Either you are not feeding me properly or you do not love me!

The Cat

The cat is a hunter, particularly independent and tough. He is born to hunt and eat mice and field mice; sometimes he brings back a small rabbit, part of a squirrel or even a bird - that's his nature! Cat owners would be well advised to give their cat enough to eat without overfeeding it! So many cats who live in houses or flats are too overweight and heavy, don't have enough space to play and are too unfit to hunt. Milk, cheese, meat and fish are the cat's preferred foods but why not give them to your cat uncooked? Indeed, in the wild, a cat fending for itself doesn't know how to cook! For the domesticated cat at home, ready-prepared tinned food and biscuits, used in the past as a "quick fix" when nothing else was available, have unfortunately now become a habit. It is still possible, when you have time, to prepare your cat's food so that it is varied and with more raw ingredients than the tinned variety. You should also give your cat the chance to catch his own food: mice from the house, field mice from cellars and outbuildings, rats ... Usually, your cat will proudly show you his prey before retreating to a quiet corner to feast on it.

The cat is an independent animal, autonomous and tough (although his immune system is rather delicate). The town cat is far more delicate than the country cat, and his main ailments will be viral, pulmonary and digestive infections, feline leucosis, bacterial infections and cutaneous problems.

We will also cover fractures and, of course, everything you need to know on the subject of nutrition to provide a well-balanced diet.

My advice

- don't overfeed your cat
- let your cat hunt: it's his natural role and gives him pleasure!
- and, of course, give your cat plenty of love and spend some time playing with him.

Feeding the cat that lives in a house or flat

- mice, if he can find any, which you should leave for him to hunt
- fish and meat
- small amounts of cheese
- milk, which he loves when he is little
- rice (to provide glucosides), vegetables
- you can also add biscuits and other prepared foods, or yeast, an excellent B group vitamin supplement which your cat will especially enjoy
- you should remember that by feeding your cat entirely on tinned food, you are not providing a healthy diet: if you fed a human being entirely on tinned food, that person would soon tire of it and their health would deteriorate. The same is true for a cat, even a domesticated one.

Giving birth

A female cat is very independent and will hide herself away (for protection) to give birth. If your cat is not very independent, prepare a clean bed for her where you can keep an eye on her. A infusion of cold sage or hydrosol of sage, or an infusion of verbena, will ease the birthing process. Add this to her food 3 to 4 days prior to the birth.

Gestation lasts 63 to 70 days.

Exhaustion, fatigue

Leave the animal to rest with water freely available - instinct tells them not to eat - for 1 to 2 days, followed by two or three small portions of food over the day, and your cat should soon be back on its feet. Add 1 to 2 drops of essential oil of orange or 1 drop of essential oil of camomile to the food for the next 2 to 3 days.

Weight loss, anaemia, anorexia

Anorexia or loss of appetite for more than 4 to 5 days warrants a visit to your vet. Add 2 to 3 drops of wild marjoram to drinking water and give yeast for 10 days.

Both male and female cats lose a lot of weight when they are mating. As long as your cat looks happy, don't panic! He will sleep and fast. Should his manner be otherwise, it could be a case of anaemia, in which case you should consult your vet. A prolonged period of anorexia can be fatal for cats.

Poisoning

The cat might eat a mouse which, in turn, has eaten rat poison (generally, a cat living in the country can detect this whilst a town cat, whose instinct has become dulled, is no longer so well informed!).

Call your vet. Your cat should be given an emetic as soon as possible.
- one drop of essential oil of mint
- administer an anal flush with the aid of a small ear syringe, for example
- make the cat swallow one tablespoon of the following solution: 20 g of magnesium chloride in 1 litre of water, then a second tablespoon one hour later, followed by an infusion of boldo or a teaspoon of castor oil which may help to induce vomiting and elimination.
- the vet should administer an appropriate antidote, particularly in the case of "chemical" poisoning.

Aromatic vermifuges

These are used to treat intestinal parasites, 1 drop twice a day for 3 days.

Constituents of vermifugal essential oils
EO of bergamot   *5 ml*
EO of sassafras   *5 ml*
EO of caraway   *5 ml*

Abscesses

1. These should be encouraged to come to a head. Apply a poultice of cabbage leaves (crush large outer leaves first) or of clay - see chapter entitled *Practical advice* - until the abscess bursts.

2. Clean with compresses and several drops of lavender. Consult your vet if you do not succeed in draining the abscess.

3. Continue the clay poultices to promote healing until the area has completely recovered.

Note

We must remember that in natural medicine, abscesses are manifestations of toxins being eliminated. We must therefore bring them to a head and not drive them back in!

Abraded pads, thorn in the paw

Cats rarely suffer from this (see *Practical advice* at the beginning of this book).

The animal has difficulty putting its paw to the ground, either as a result of walking a long way over gravel or stones, in which case the trauma is due to *abraded pads*, or because of a thorn or a splinter lodged between the claws, or even a spikelet (known in Provence as *espigaü*).

In both cases, a clay poultice should be applied until the condition improves and the foreign body has been eliminated. Alternate the poultice with a blend of St John's wort oil and EO of lavender. (Key aromatic blend A.)

Fleas

Fleas are enemies of cats as much as they are of dogs. Unfortunately, cats do not appreciate essential oils at all and their particularly sensitive skin cannot tolerate them. A good solution is to cover your cat's bed with mint leaves or lavender seed, which fleas detest. You can also render the area aseptic by using a diffusion of Freshtonic*, which often drives fleas away.

* Product of Laboratoire Vie'Arôme, 13690 - Graveson-en-Provence, France

Coughs, emphysema

Generally, it is only cats that are overfed or incorrectly fed that develop coughs. Treatment is relatively simple: the cat's instinct tells it not to eat, but only to drink.
- put on a diet of water only for 1 to 2 days
- administer a vermifuge
- place an aromatic diffuser containing respiratory essential oils in your cat's living area.

In special circumstances, such as a stay at the vet's, for example, the cat should be put in a cage with respiratory essential oils once or twice a day for 15 minutes.

If the cage is of the enclosed rather than the open design, place the diffuser inside for 5 minutes and the leave the cat there for a further 5 minutes. Repeat this 4 or 5 times daily.

NEVER MASSAGE A CAT WITH ESSENTIAL OILS!
The cat may breathe them in, but his fur and skin cannot tolerate them.

Respiratory essential oils blend for the diffuser
EO of eucalyptus	*20 ml*
EO of pine	*10 ml*
EO of tea-tree	*5 ml*
EO of thyme	*2 ml*

Use as it is in an aromatic diffuser.

Or just use essential oil of eucalyptus, the finest of the respiratory essential oils, on its own.

Coryza, typhus

These infectious diseases, serious and even fatal in cats, respond very well to an aromatic treatment, and easily substitute for traditional antibiotics.

In this case, the essential oils for the aromatogram*[1] are chosen for their fast-acting efficiency: essential oil of wild marjoram, thyme, lemon, mint, coriander, cinnamon and savory. The aromatogram test will almost certainly bring up one of these.

Of course, your vet can recommend an aromatogram just as he would a antibiogram*[2] - it's up to you to make it clear that you prefer a treatment using essential oils!

Notes
*[1] "Aromatogram": a combination of specifically chosen essential oils, the sum of which has greater and differing properties than each constituent essential oil.
*[2] "Antibiogram": similar to the "aromatogram", but using traditional medicine, specifically dependant on antibiotics and painkilling drugs.

Fractures

The vet will either set the broken bone in plaster, or use a splint or pin, to be left in place for several weeks. As soon as the plaster has been removed, you can speed up the healing of the broken bone with clay poultices.

To prepare a clay poultice

Take either a tube of ready-to-use clay or dissolve clay powder in a little water until you obtain a "bread dough" consistency.

Apply clay a good centimetre thick on to a double layer of gauze and place on the damaged limb - the gauze allows removal of the clay without pulling the fur.

The poultice should be left on for 1 to 3 hours in the morning and evening for approximately a week.

To make the clay paste, use a glass or earthenware (not plastic or metal) dish and mix with a wooden (not metal) spoon.

To activate the clay, place it in the sun for several hours before use.

During this period, you should supplement the cat's diet with ½ teaspoon per day of wheat germ oil (natural vitamin E) and 1 tablespoon per day of yeast (B vitamins).

The clay poultices will help the broken bone to knit together much faster, just as they do for human bones.

Cat odours

The best way to eliminate cat odours is to use a diffusion of purifying essential oils that have a strong, fresh smell. Of all the aromatic blends we have tried, the following, called Freshtonic*, satisfies the greatest number of users and is not disliked by cats.

To eliminate the odour of cat urine:

Freshtonic 2
EO of lavender	*30 ml*
EO of mint	*5 ml*
EO of lemon	*10 ml*
EO of terebinth	*15 ml*

For use in the diffuser just as it is.

You can also make up the following blend:
EO of pine	*50 ml*
EO of mint	*10 ml*

or else use lavender and mint, or terebinth, pine and mint. Essential oil of eucalyptus is not sufficient to hide the smell of cat urine; essential oil of exotic verbena repels cats; none of the mild essential oils mixes well with cat odours.

The respiratory essential oils (see special blend above) are equally effective in eliminating cat odours.

These principal odour problems can thus be resolved using essential oils which, we should not forget, are all antiseptic in their action.

* *Laboratoire Vie'Arôme - 13690 Graveson-en-Provence, France*

To summarise

Our friend the cat must not be abandoned at holiday times, needs to be loved and well treated, and not overfed. We should give it plenty of attention - it will more than repay us with its companionship, cooperation and loyalty.

In the rare cases where more specific treatment is required, you can refer to another book by the same author, *Aromatherapy from Provence*; for cats, divide all dosages for internal treatment by 3. Above all, never use essential oil massage on cats - their sensitive skin cannot tolerate the essential oils!

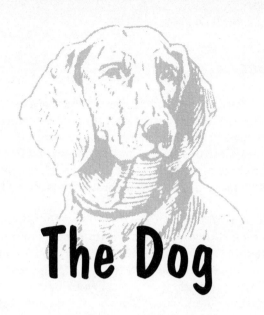

The Dog

The dog's prayer

Once I am born, you will choose me and look after me for life
And if I forget myself sometimes in the house, forgive me, I am still only young.
You will see that when I am grown up I'll be clean and sensible.
I will ask of you almost nothing, only a little affection and a crust of bread.
In exchange, I will guard your property and never let anyone bother you.
My love and loyalty for you will grow
And you will be my universe, my future and my joy.
You will be my lord and master; I will be your slave and your child.
Without hesitation, I will give my life for you; but please, I beseech you, never abandon me!
Never abandon me!

The Dog

Man's faithful friend, companion to the traveller and the shepherd, and solace to the lonely, or simply bringer of joy, the dog runs, hunts, searches, enjoys life - and revels in the freedom of nature. Dogs are not made to live in the confined space of a house or flat, but if this is the case, then two long walks a day are indispensable for their well-being.

To give dogs the respect we owe them, there are several golden rules to follow which, unfortunately, are sometimes forgotten: never ill-treat or hit your dog; don't abandon it when you go on holiday (or when you come back!). If you find a lost or abandoned dog, do your best to reunite it with its owner (look under "Lost or Abandoned" listings in the small ads); for the owners of bitches, puppies initially given a home should be given away or sold as soon as one knows that one cannot keep them; dogs need attention, care and food every day; love, play and time devoted to the animal are fundamental to their happiness. Our grandparents used to prepare the dogs' supper using leftovers from the evening meal, both raw and cooked, mixed with water and ground rice or meal (made from whole cereals) and the dogs were never overfed!

Dogs naturally purge their systems if they live outside and in the country: when they are out, they will carefully choose those specific plants they need. When a dog becomes "civilised", it loses this instinct and needs to be purged more often.

The dog living in the country also likes to eat fruit growing on trees, such as apples, pears and cherries, and even blackberries and raspberries from the bushes. If your dog crunches carrots when it is young, it will continue to enjoy raw carrots.

Of course, dogs are hunters, and it is not unlikely that you will see your dog come back one day triumphantly carrying a chicken or a duck to show to any puppies there may be: a female dog will display and provide the most suitable food for her puppies. It is therefore up to us, their owners, to give our dogs whatever they need to prevent havoc in the neighbouring henhouse!

The ultra-civilised dog who lives in town will be more susceptible to illness in general, its resistance being lower.

Feeding your dog

Large or small, dogs are faithful friends and always considerate towards us. In return, we should take special care with their food.

Generally, there are many ready-made dog foods available; however, you will need to add some supplements to these.

- *yeast*: rich in natural B group vitamins, it's good for the coat, enhances energy levels and helps to prevent dermatoses. Furthermore, yeast has a taste similar to cheese, and dogs love it.

- *wheat germ oil*: rich in natural vitamin B, this is excellent for bone formation and the nervous system. Can be used periodically as a three-week curative treatment, mainly for puppies and elderly or infirm animals.

- dogs need *raw beef bones* or veal bones (never rabbit bones) and *raw meat*, both for play and for their general health; these are genuine treats, unlike sugar, which is a real 'poison' for dogs.

- *raw and/or cooked vegetables* should also be an integral part of your dog's diet. If you prepare vegetable or carrot juice for yourself, mix the discarded peelings from the juicer with the yeast that you add to the food. Even if the dog is used only to cooked vegetables, add a small amount of raw vegetables in with the cooked.

- our canine friends adore *vegetable oils* such as those in leftover salad dressings, provided these contain no vinegar or lemon juice.

- don't forget that most country dogs are very fond of eating fruits and berries that they come across on trees and bushes in the course of their wanderings. They also enjoy nuts and dried fruit!

Watch your dog's weight just as you would your own; don't overfeed your dog. An obese dog will be more susceptible to illness and infections.

To summarise

Dogs need as natural a diet as possible: meat, bones and vegetables, or ready-prepared croquettes only if you cannot do otherwise, in which case you should add every day:

- yeast, to make up 10% of the daily ration.
- wheat germ or wheat germ oil as a treatment lasting 3 weeks, given 3 or 4 times a year.

These simple dietary steps will ensure that your dog has enhanced resistance to disease, as well as improved mental and physical well-being.

If you cannot prepare your dog's food personally, ask your vet to supply you with dog food specifically intended for your dog, to which you can add the supplements listed above.

Pregnancy

To the standard diet, you should add a double ration of wheat germ oil (vitamin E), half a teaspoon per day for every 20 kg of body weight.

In addition, the mother-to-be will crave more raw meat, bones, cheese rind, eggs and olive oil.

Yeast is recommended of course, but this should already form part of her daily diet.

Giving birth

Bitches used to the freedom of the countryside will choose a spot in the garden that they have already prepared several hours previously in which to give birth, and it is generally one that is away from prying eyes.

> *Tara, a Beauce shepherd, 6 years old, chose a spot underneath a huge laurel bush in which to give birth, then she carried her puppies each day to other bushes, either bamboo, thuja or another laurel.*

Town dogs accept the place that is offered to them, seeking out the warmth of the basket provided for the purpose in the house or kennel.

Several days before the event, your dog will either be feverish and overexcited or quiet and passive. Meanwhile, line a large basket with newspapers and blankets, that way she will have a choice of location. Give her plenty of water, adding 1 to 2 tablespoons of hydrosol of sage to her drinking water for 3 or 4 days before labour is due, or an infusion of verbena. If she is overexcited, add 3 or 4 drops of essential oil of lavender or orange (see feeding during pregnancy).

Gestation lasts 57 to 60 days.

Suckling

You shouldn't forget to provide more water than usual, a little milk, one or two eggs per day, some fennel juice, some wheat germ oil, some olive oil, some yeast, and above all, remember to double her usual food ration.

While she is still suckling, it is a good idea to add some pureed raw carrots or fresh vegetable juices to her food; two meals a day will be welcomed, and will not make her unduly fat: she needs to be slim and alert during this period of overexertion. Some easily absorbed calcium (oligo trace elements) or other food supplements will be most beneficial during her pregnancy.

When she has finished suckling, her diet can gradually be returned to normal. It would be advisable to give her a purgative and a vermifuge* at the end of suckling, to cleanse the internal system.

Note
* Vermifuge: any drug or chemical agent used to expel worms from the intestine.

Feeding the puppies

Just as for a human baby, solid food should be gradually introduced as suckling diminishes; the mother's milk, or a substitute milk if the mother has none or has been separated from the puppy, remains the most important food.

A puppy is normally weaned at around two months.

Puppies should receive three to four meals per day during their second and third months, and then two meals per day from four to six months, depending on what your vet advises.

Our grandparents used to give puppies enriched so-called "hen's milk", which was actually cow's milk with added egg and honey (the honey being optional), or reconstituted bitch's milk (consisting of egg, sugar and cow's milk - although I recommend honey rather than sugar).

To this enriched milk you could add yeast, bearing in mind that now is the time to gradually start introducing pieces of raw meat (minced, to start with, depending on the size of dog).

At this point you can also add some raw carrot juice (or grated carrots), so as to get the puppy used to raw foods, which are healthier and provide more energy. Wheat germ oil should be added to the daily diet: it is an excellent source of vitamin E, good for growth, bone formation and the protection of the nervous system.

Pureed cereals are often added to milk for babies in the first few months. Personally, I prefer to enrich the milk with yeast.

To summarise

- the famous "hen's milk" that our grandparents used to prepare is still useful today: milk with eggs and sugar (or, better still, honey).
- raw carrots (or carrots pureed in the blender), to which has been added yeast and enriched milk. Gradually, cereals and raw meat can be introduced.
- puppy treats: raw veal bones to gnaw - a favourite food and plaything - and, of course, yeast.

The "domesticated" dog should be given his usual balanced diet (special milk for puppies) with the addition of the items indicated above.

Vaccinations

For or against? Everyone is free to choose and your natural therapy vet will be able to advise you.

If your dog travels with you when you go away, an anti-rabies vaccine is compulsory for certain places. Up-to-date information is available from your vet.

You may like to know that there are homoeopathic vaccines available for dogs (although these are not officially recognized and do not entitle you to the appropriate stamp on the vaccination record).

Some vets will prescribe, in addition to vaccines, complementary homoeopathic remedies to counteract the harmful effects of a traditional vaccine.

We should remember that a dog that is well fed and cared for (with the quality foods, essential oils and food supplements previously indicated) will have a significantly enhanced resistance to disease. Pasteur and/or Claude Bernard would have said: "The microbe is nothing, the 'soil' is all". This conclusion challenges a lifetime's work and research. Just as with the human, the "soil" and its degree of resistance depend principally on its nutrition.

Worms

Worming should be carried out every three months in puppies under a year, then once or twice a year thereafter. Worming should form part of your dog's basic case routine.

You can choose between a traditional worming product recommended by your vet, or the following mixture which you can give either in a capsule, if your dog is fussy, or simply add to his food. Whichever method you choose, vermifugal essential oils are effective on worm-infested soil, resulting in a reduction and perhaps even the avoidance of the need for traditional worming treatments for dogs raised healthily from birth and accustomed to aromatic treatments.

Before worming a dog with an aromatic vermifuge, it is advisable to administer a purgative.

Natural aromatic vermifuge
Essential oils of bergamot, caraway, sassafras, wild marjoram and thyme, in equal parts.

Mix all ingredients together in a bottle. Give 5 drops twice a day for 3 days per 10 kg of body weight, giving a large dog, weighing 60 kg for example, 30 drops per day.

Magnesium chloride treatment
Use 20 g of magnesium chloride per litre of water, to make 1 litre of this mixture.

Give 1 tablespoon per day for every 10 kg of body weight for 10 days, at each change of season, which corresponds to one glass a day for a dog of 50 or 60 kg.

Magnesium chloride also strengthens the natural immune system against parasites.

Worming

If your dog continues to suffer from worms, I would recommend that you administer a purgative, followed by an aromatic vermifuge.

Essential oil of garlic is an excellent vermifuge (2 drops twice a day for a dog of 20 kg (especially good for tape worm). However, essential oil of garlic is often difficult to administer because of its strong, unpleasant odour. You can also give your dog raw garlic, just as for horses.

Exhaustion

After a long hunt or a strenuous sexual encounter, our friend the dog may be exhausted. Rest, calm and a starvation diet for 24 to 48 hours, with plenty of water to drink, is the answer. Your dog's natural instinct will be to purge its system by eating certain plants, if it lives in the country. When you reintroduce food, divide the daily ration into two or three smaller portions. Add 1 to 3 drops, depending on the animal's weight, of essential oil of orange to the drinking water for 48 hours, then provide 1 to 3 drops of essential oil of rosemary or coriander for the next week.

If your dog does not recover after this treatment, you should consult your vet.

Fatigue

Essential oils will be of great benefit to a dog that is tired and mournful, and it should be back on form within a few days.

Essential oil blend to counteract fatigue in dogs
EO of rosemary	*10 ml*
EO of rose geranium	*5 ml*
EO of cinnamon	*2 ml*
EO of coriander	*3 ml*

Give twice a day for 5 to 10 days, 1 drop of the mixture per 10 kg of body weight.

You can also use approximately 20 drops of the same mixture as a massage on the neck and stomach, twice a day.

In cases of chronic fatigue, you can also administer a magnesium chloride treatment (see p 52).

Weight loss, anaemia, anorexia

Anorexia or "loss of appetite" for more than 4 or 5 days warrants a visit to the vet. Add 2 or 3 drops of wild marjoram to drinking water and give extra yeast for 10 days.

Where there is weight loss outside the mating season, something unusual is going on if the animal seems sad and you should consult your vet as it could be a case of anaemia.

If the animal has lost weight but otherwise seems happy, don't panic! It might take a few days to get back to normal, but there's nothing to worry about.

Poisoning

In cases of emergency, call the vet immediately then administer an emetic or an enema, according to your practitioner's instructions.

Following this, give 1 drop of essential oil of mint every hour for 5 to 6 hours.

In cases of "chemical" poisoning, an antidote is necessary.

In any case, you can add a magnesium chloride treatment (see page 52) during the 3 weeks after the specific "poisoning" treatment.

Purgatives

If you choose an essential oil vermifuge, the purgative should be magnesium or *Chlorumagène* (a proprietary laxative lotion based on magnesium).

Give one teaspoon of one of these for every 10 kg of body weight, twice a day for 3 days.

Purgatives have traditionally been incorporated into allopathic vermifuges.

A castor oil purgative can be used to flush out the system more thoroughly in cases of poor digestion, rheumatism or paralysis, and can be alternated with magnesium or *Chlorumagène* over 3 days. The dosage is one tablespoon per 10 kg of body weight.

Bacterial and other infectious diseases

Whatever the precise cause, the same treatment applies:
the essential oils indicated by the aromatogram
or the formula for the APH* blend:
*EOs of thyme, cinnamon, coriander, clove, nutmeg, pine,
savory and ylang-ylang, to which should be added an equal
volume of EO of wild marjoram (origanum vulgare).*
Use 3 drops of the mixture 3 times a day per 10 kg of body
weight.

Introduce a magnesium chloride treatment (20 g per litre of
water, one tablespoon per 10 kg of body weight, twice a
day). In animals, magnesium chloride stimulates the natural
immune system and increases resistance to disease.

Also, an aromatic diffuser providing the following oils can
be used continuously:
Makes 100 ml:

EO of lavandin	*40 ml*
EO of thyme	*10 ml*
EO of wild marjoram	*10 ml*
EO of eucalyptus	*20 ml*
EO of mint	*5 ml*
EO of cinnamon	*5 ml*
EO of rosemary	*10 ml*

* APH is one of the aromatic body oil blends, specifically to
enhance mental alertness, physical equilibrium, memory,
sexual drive and cellular vitality (action).

Abscesses

1. You should allow the abscess to come to a head. Apply a cabbage leaf poultice (crush the outer leaves first) or a clay poultice (see *Practical advice*) until the abscess bursts naturally.

2. Clean and empty the abscess site (often a foreign body needs to be removed, and this comes out easily with a clay poultice). Add several drops of essential oil of lavender to the cleansing compress.

3. Alternate clay poultices with compresses of essential oil of lavender mixed with oil of St John's wort until the site has healed completely.

Abraded pads, thorn in the paw

When the animal has difficulty putting its paw to the ground, this may be either as a result of walking a long way over gravel or stones, in which case the trauma is due to *abraded pads*, or because of a thorn or a splinter or even a spikelet (known in Provence as an *espigaü*) between the claws (see *Practical advice* at the beginning of the book).

In both cases, a clay poultice should be applied until the condition improves and the foreign body is eliminated. Alternate the poultice with a blend of St John's wort oil and essential oil of lavender.

Fractures

The vet will either apply a pin or a splint or set the bone in plaster, depending on the seriousness of the fracture.

To ease the treatment, you can add a clay poultice, which speeds up bone remodelling. This should also be done if the vet cannot be consulted immediately.

How do you make a clay poultice?

Take some pieces of clay and mix with water in a glass or earthenware bowl using a wooden spoon; do not let the clay come into contact with any metal or plastic object. When the mixture is thick and smooth, place a 2 cm thick layer onto gauze and apply to the wound, fastening with a bandage or strip of material. You can apply the clay directly to the skin, but some of the fur will be pulled off when the poultice is removed. Leave the clay poultice on for at least 3 hours then renew it, and continue doing this over the next 2 or 3 weeks, which is the approximate time it takes for the fracture to heal.

During this period, give your dog extra "raw" food in his diet: meat and vegetables, no sugar or cheese, and, of course, extra yeast (2 large tablespoons per day for every 10 kg of body weight), wheat germ oil (1 teaspoon per day) and magnesium chloride treatment (20 g per litre of water, about half a glass twice a day added to drinking water or food - magnesium chloride is very salty).

If you want to improve the quality of the clay, and reactivate it, simply place it in the sun for several hours before use.

Rheumatism

Just like humans, many dogs suffer from rheumatism as they get older.

Rheumatoid and osteoarthritic symptoms often result from overfeeding, lack of exercise or hereditary disorders. In dogs, rapid intervention is necessary before the onset of ankylosis or even total or partial paralysis, principally of the hind-quarters in the first instance.

The second possible cause of rheumatism can be a vertebral blockage, which the osteopathic vet will be able to put right easily.

What can I do?
- reduce daily quantity of food
- replace by raw and cooked vegetables: pureed carrot pulp, grated carrots or carrot juice, mixed with yeast, for approximately a week
- during this week, administer a purgative daily: magnesium *san pellegrino* (1 tablespoon per 20 kg of body weight)
- give plenty of water, of course - your dog will have a tendency to drink much more
- for delicate animals, such as Yorkshire terriers, purgatives should be introduced very gradually.

As an aromatherapy treatment, add to the daily diet (i.e., the pureed carrots with added yeast) 1 drop of juniper essential oil and 1 drop of birch essential oil per 10 kg of body weight.

To treat locally, you can massage morning and evening with the following essential oils:

Essential oils blend for antirheumatic massage
Mix together 10 ml each of essential oil of pine, thyme, rosemary, terebinth, birch and juniper and add to 60 ml of oil of St John's wort.

Massage the stomach area generally with the mixture, using about 20 drops directly on the affected parts.

Within 3 or 4 days, your dog's suffering will have been alleviated; you should continue the treatment, however, for at least a week.

Revert to a normal, healthy diet, as detailed in the section entitled *Feeding*, whilst continuing with the massage morning and evening.

You can repeat the emergency treatment described above for one week every month until the symptoms have disappeared.

Note
If your dog has a very painful joint, a clay poultice is always welcome - see the section on *Fractures*.

Don't forget to consult an osteopathic vet in these situations!

Paralysis

Elderly dogs and cats who have been overfed can suffer from paralysis (see section on *Rheumatism*).

At the beginning of the attack: put dog on a starvation diet for 2 to 3 days with plenty of water to drink, to which you should add 2 tablespoons of hydrosol of juniper or elder per litre.

Administer a purgative to the dog using castor oil (see *Purgatives* p 52): this often works like magic!

An antirheumatic massage can be given to the hind-quarters or other paralysed part twice a day.

The application of clay poultices can usefully complete this treatment.

Skin diseases and dermatoses

The king of all remedies is still magnesium chloride: half a glass of a solution made up with 20 g magnesium chloride per litre of water, given twice a day.

Another remedy consists of adding yeast to the food, which should, in fact, be part of the daily routine.

A third possible remedy consists of applying the following mixture twice a day:
1. *hydrosol of cedar, thyme and lavender*
2. *EO of terebinth, lavender and pine in equal parts.*
Apply these mixtures at regular intervals until complete recovery.

These three treatments are equally effective for loss of fur, eczema and almost all dermatoses.

In the case of eczema, it is very important to eliminate all sweet things from the diet, those delicacies that we like to give to our dog as a treat and which are in fact a poison to him!

In addition to the blend of essential oils given above, we can add a second formula:
essential oils of rose geranium, rosewood, pine and lavender, in equal parts, mixed with the same volume of oils of St John's wort and wheat germ.

Ticks

We all know how important it is when removing ticks to ensure the removal of the whole body of these unpleasant creatures. Don't forget to burn them afterwards, otherwise cats and dogs can easily pick them up again. You should also be sure to clean the bedding, the cushions, the kennel and the house - yes, ticks have even been known to climb walls! There are many commercial products available.

Anti-tick aromatic blend (makes 1 litre)
EO of terebinth	*500 ml*
EO of lavender or lavandin	*100 ml*
Oil of St John's wort	*100 ml*
Olive oil	*300 ml*

Massage the affected parts gently with the mixture. The ticks will drop out immediately and over the next 10 minutes or so. Burn them.

As a preventative measure, especially in summer, massage the stomach area, the fold of the thigh, behind the ears, and around the eyes, with this mixture once a week.

Fleas

The flea is the No. 1 enemy of dogs. An insidious creature, it not only hides in the dog's fur, but also in carpets, floor coverings and old parquet.

Many anti-flea remedies are available, ranging from collars (which are often poorly tolerated) to powders, shampoos and lotions, but these should only be used on the advice of your vet.

Otherwise, here are a few aromatic remedies:

1. - EO of terebinth   *½ volume*
     olive oil or 90% alcohol   *½ volume*

2. - EO of mint   *¼ volume*
     olive oil or 90% alcohol   *¾ volume*

3. - A layer of mint left in the dog's bedding (fleas dislike mint)

4. - EO of lemongrass (especially in tropical countries)

The flea can transmit pulicosis, a type of eczema associated with fur loss and itching, that may become infected. Prevention is therefore more important than cure - as we all know, anyway.

The secret of a beautiful coat

Dogs need B group vitamin supplements, present in yeast that should be added regularly to their food.

Rubbing the coat with essential oil of terebinth (use a good quality oil, not like the turpentine used for painting or cleaning purposes) will keep it healthy and glossy.

However, it is the good and healthy nutrition, discussed earlier, which is the principle cause of a good coat (see Nutrition page 38).

To prevent fetid breath

2 drops of a mixture of essential oils of caraway, cumin and coriander should be added daily to the food.

If the dog will accept it, 2 drops of essential oil of mint can also be added once or twice a day.

In addition, it is recommended that you have your dog's teeth cleaned regularly at the vet's.

To summarise

We have seen how important a role diet plays in the health and happiness of all our canine friends, large and small.

In addition to a balanced diet, worming and food supplements are also necessary for both town and country dogs.

Daily exercise and fresh air, bones to gnaw, and cutting down on sweet things, are all sensible practices to follow.

Finally, in connection with the central focus of this book, essential oils can be used, just as in humans, both as a preventative measure and as a treatment whenever it is considered necessary, either as a massage or as a dietary supplement.

The use of aromatic diffusers, with their antiseptic, respiratory and balsamic blends, should be used in the treatment of infectious, respiratory problems, and odour problems.

The speed of action and efficiency of essential oils means that they work extremely well with other natural therapies such as homoeopathy and osteopathy by ensuring in every case that toxins are eliminated and that the disease is not suppressed. Essential oils, clay and purgatives are simple and effective treatments for shock.

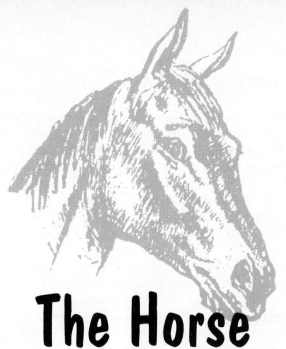

The Horse

The horse's prayer

I submit my prayer to you, Master.
Feed me, quench my thirst and, after the day's work is
over, give me a clean, healthy stable.
Talk to me - the voice is more effective than the whip,
teach me to work willingly and try to understand me
without mistreating me.
Take care that my feet are not damaged by ill-fitting
shoes, and if I seem to be off my food, check my
teeth. Don't cut my mane or my tail, they are my only
defence against the flies.
Dear Master, when I grow feeble or infirm with age,
spare me suffering, and take pity on me.
Finally, forgive me for approaching you with this
humble prayer in the name of He who, after all, was
born in a stable.

The horse

Whether a horse is a walking companion, or in a training or racing environment, the animal requires a great deal of attention both in terms of food and general management. The box or stable should be clean and healthy, the diet must be in direct relation to the amount of physical work expected of the animal (racing, pulling loads, labouring), and its coat and feet must be kept in good condition - all these demand daily prevention and care.

The main problems that vets and animal breeders come across in stables are: lameness, abscesses of a bony, tendinous, articular or muscular origin, cardiovascular problems, pulmonary problems (coughs, emphysema ...), intestinal parasites, stress (particularly in race horses), dermatoses and problems of gait.

In all these instances, essential oils will improve resistance to disease by increasing the animal's vitality and allowing the elimination of accumulated toxins.

Essential oils can be used:
- internally
- as a massage
- by diffusion into the atmosphere.

Regular use of the diffuser with a purifying or respiratory blend provides all the benefits of aromatic essential oils, thereby avoiding the effects of chills in working horses.

Regular use of essential oils either for a specific problem or to maintain a high level of vitality generally, maximises the horse's resistance to disease and its performance in general.

Feeding racehorses

Grains and oats, hay, carrots and apples, no white sugar, plenty of water, and ...
daily food supplements of:
- wheat germ oil (E vitamins), 1 tablespoon
- yeast (B vitamins), 5 to 10 tablespoons
- cold-pressed oil, made from the first pressing (olive, sunflower, sesame, safflower)
- garlic, onion, cabbage, beetroot, egg, potatoes, soya ...
- HAY (you can never give them enough!) preferably organically grown.

Avoid white sugar - cane sugar or unrefined sugar beet are preferable.

For one week per month, add to the drinking water one glass daily of magnesium chloride solution at a concentration of 20 g per litre of water. The magnesium chloride increases resistance to disease by strengthening the immune system and reducing the effects of stress.

For 10 days every month, give a calcium treatment in the form of calcium carbonate (3 to 4 heaped tablespoons).

For 1 week per month give a tonic blend of essential oils:
- *EO of rosemary*   *10ml*
- *EO of eucalyptus*   *5ml*
- *EO of coriander*   *5ml*
- *EO of nutmeg*   *5ml*

Blend together in 60ml of wheat germ oil.
Give 90 drops once a day, for 7 days each month.

Stress, anxiety and nervous tics

Stress in horses can be the result of too much racing, hereditary factors, or even a lack of grass or hay ("*fodder deficiency*": in this latter case, the horse doesn't chew enough and stress builds up!). The following essential oils help combat stress in horses and promote mental well-being and nervous equilibrium.

They can be used in three ways: taken internally, by massage and by diffusion into the atmosphere.

For internal treatment, use 10 drops twice a day for 3 to 6 weeks. This can be added to food gradually so the horse gets used to the particular odour of the essential oils.

Two "Anti-stress" essential oil blends, to be taken internally

Formula 1
EO of lavender	15 ml
EO of sweet marjoram	10 ml
EO of basil	5 ml
EO of verbena	2 ml

Blend together in 60 ml of wheat germ oil and give 30 drops twice a day.

Formula 2
EO of lavender	15 ml
EO of sweet marjoram	5 ml
EO of bitter orange leaves	5 ml
Eo of neroli	1 ml
EO of orange	10 ml
EO of verbena	1 ml

Mix together in 60 ml of wheat germ oil and give 30 drops twice a day.

"Anti-stress" essential oil massage blend

EO of lavender	40 ml
EO of sweet marjoram	30 ml
EO of basil	10 ml
EO of bitter orange leaves	18 ml
EO of neroli	2 ml

Mix together in 200 ml of sesame or soya oil and massage once a day from head to tail via the belly.

"Anti-stress" essential oil blend for diffusers

EO of lavender	30 ml
EO of sweet marjoram	20 ml
EO of bitter orange	20 ml
EO of pine	28 ml
EO of verbena	1 ml
EO of neroli	0.5 ml

Place in diffuser without any other mix and use it daily. Especially good for race horses.

Stress in horses is often due to inappropriate living conditions. Like any other country animal or animal in service, the horse needs love or ... freedom.

Abscesses

Most abscesses, if badly managed, lead to lameness, which causes suffering to the animal and is unacceptable, particularly where the horse is kept for showing or racing. It is preferable to treat abscesses by natural means rather than administer excessively powerful anti-inflammatory injections.

1. You should allow the abscess to come to a head. Apply a cabbage leaf poultice (crush the large outer leaves first) or a clay poultice (see section entitled *Practical advice*) until the abscess bursts naturally.

2. Clean and empty the abscess site (often a foreign body needs to be removed, and this comes out easily with a clay poultice). Add several drops of essential oil of lavender to the cleansing compress.

3. Continue to alternate clay poultices with compresses of essential oil of lavender mixed with oil of St John's wort until the site has healed completely.

Worming

Horses should be wormed at least every two months. Worming is very specific - your homoeopathic or natural therapy vet will be well acquainted with aromatherapy practices that are used to strengthen natural resistance in an environment where worm infestation is common.

Aromatic worming blend

EO of bergamot	*15 ml*
EO of caraway	*15 ml*
EO of wild marjoram	*10 ml*
EO of sassafras	*20 ml*

Add 5 drops of the mixture three times a day to the food or ask your pharmacist to make up the mixture into capsules and give 3 capsules a day for 3 days.

Added regularly to food, garlic also helps to control worms permanently. The remarkable "worming" properties of garlic are available in its raw vegetable form, so it is not necessary to use the essential oil of garlic.

Coughs and respiratory problems

Whether used in diffusion, as a massage or taken internally, respiratory essential oils promote expectoration and soothe irritation. Massage with the palm of the hand on the chest and throat once or twice a day during periods of attacks; 1 tablespoon per massage is sufficient for a horse. In diffusion: use an electric diffuser in the stall for 1 or 2 hours per day. During periods of attack, leave the diffuser on all day and administer two massages daily.

Respiratory essential oil blend to use as a massage

EO of eucalyptus	30 ml
EO of lavender	15 ml
EO of pine	20 ml
EO of thyme	5 ml
EO of rosemary	10 ml
Eo of terebinth	15 ml
EO of cinnamon	2 ml
EO of wild marjoram	3 ml

This massage remedy can be used just as it is or diluted in sesame, soya or olive oil. If you use it in diffusion in the stall, it is essential to use it undiluted or else use one of the following respiratory remedies:

1.
EO of pine	30ml
EO of thyme	10ml
EO of fir	15ml
EO of tea-tree	10ml
EO of orange	15ml
EO of terebinth	30ml

2.
EO of pine	40ml
EO of eucalyptus	40ml
EO of thyme	10ml
EO of terebinth	20ml

3. *EO of eucalyptus (niaouli or cajeput)*   *40ml*
   EO of lavandin   *40ml*
   EO of pine   *20ml*

In all cases of coughing, worming is recommended at the beginning of aromatic treatment as some coughs are fundamentally the result of a parasitic infestation.

Aches and muscular pains

Essential oils promote warm-up and aid recovery after exertion; they prevent general aches and pains and inflammation of tendons.

Essential oils can be used as a massage before exercise, training or a race.

In cases of chronic muscular pains, essential oils can be used twice a day until the problem is cured.

"Muscular pain" essential oil blend

EO of cinnamon	5 ml
EO of coriander	10 ml
EO of nutmeg	10 ml
EO of rosemary	20 ml
EO of lavender	10 ml
EO of pine	10 ml
EO of terebinth	20 ml
(pure, not essence of turpentine from the chemist)	
EO of white birch	10 ml
EO of verbena	5 ml

Add 100 ml of essential oils to 200 ml of oil of St John's wort, and apply to affected parts.

Joint pain, rheumatism, stiffness and lameness

The following essential oils soothe pain without treating the underlying problem - they provide only temporary relief. To promote sleep and aid recovery during rest, it would be preferable to administer them at night. During the day, it is better not to treat the pain since, in this case, it acts as a protection against excessive exercise. A racehorse with a limp or a bad foot where the pain has been completely suppressed will tend to work, run and gallop as usual, as he no longer feels pain, and the obligatory period of rest will be violated and recovery take longer as a result!

"Joint pain" aromatic blend
EO of white birch	20 ml
EO of juniper	20 ml
EO of sweet marjoram	10 ml
EO of pine	10 ml
EO of rosemary	20 ml
EO of terebinth*	10 ml
EO of lavender	10 ml

Mix 100 ml of the essential oils with 200 ml of oil of St John's wort*

* Note: essential oil of terebinth and oil of St John's wort - see section entitled *Care and regrowth of the coat*.
This blend can be massaged in, using a circular movement on the affected parts, twice a day for 3 weeks, then 3 to 4 times a year as a curative treatment thereafter.

Always use high quality essential oils that are pure and natural and not reconstituted.

During this period, take care with the animal's diet: reduce grains, which cause overheating, and provide more raw vegetables. The addition of food supplements in the form of ionised metals that can be directly assimilated is also necessary (consult your vet).

In addition to external treatment, you can give an internal treatment: 10 drops of the following mixture twice a day for a period of 3 weeks, mixed in with food gradually in such a way that the horse gets used to the odour of the oils.

"Joint pains" aromatic blend for internal treatment (makes 60 ml):

EO of pine	5 ml
EO of sweet thyme	5 ml
EO of rosemary	10 ml
EO of terebinth	10 ml
EO of white birch	15 ml
EO of juniper	15 ml

For best results, mix this with 10 times its volume of wheat germ, olive, safflower or sesame oil; and give one tablespoon of the mixture, twice a day.

Congestion, poor circulation and recovery after exertion

The following essential oils improve blood circulation, prevent bruising, windgall and congestion.

They can be used after exercise on the limbs, coronet of the hoof, pastern and fetlock, the phalanges (massage upwards), and in the hollow of the frog. Apply a few drops of the mixture to bare hands and rub in. This essential oil blend is a "comforting" one and can be used regularly. For best results, use after dousing the limbs in cold water. This remedy also helps to prevent problems of cracks in the skin at the elbow of the pastern. If a horse works irregularly, this blend helps to prevent congestion resulting from exercise or work.

Special "anti-congestion" essential oil blend

EO of rosewood	10 ml
EO of white birch	15 ml
EO of cypress	30 ml
EO of lavender	10 ml
EO of mint	5 ml
EO of sage	5 ml
EO of clary sage	5 ml

Mix together with 200 ml of oil of St John's wort and massage the legs with one tablespoon of the blend twice a day.

Note: Oil of St John's wort has two specific properties - it improves blood circulation in general and has the ability to reconstitute intervertebral cartilage (Docteur Breuss, 1920, Germany). In addition, it is an ideal active support medium for the majority of essential oils, such as wheat germ oil.

Inflammation and skin irritation

of the teat, between the legs, at the elbow of the pastern, in the axilla and at the junction of the forelimb and the shoulder

This essential oil blend can be applied locally once a day, using the palm of the hand, until the irritation subsides.

The dosage is one tablespoon in total for all the parts to be treated. Thereafter, as a maintenance dose, repeat this application once a month. In summer, you can use it before taking the horse out, on a regular basis if the animal is very sensitive to irritants.

This aromatic blend prevents irritation.
It helps to strengthen the tissues by reducing the risk of teat infection. In addition, it is an excellent decongestant for blocked teats.

"Inflammation and irritation" essential oil blend
EO of rosewood   30 ml
EO of lemon   30 ml
EO of lavender   40 ml

Mix with 50 ml of wheat germ oil, 50 ml of oil of St John's wort and 100 ml of sesame oil.

The therapeutic properties of essential oils include their antiseptic, anti-infectious and revitalising qualities. The oils can always be used in three main ways: by diffusion into the atmosphere, as a massage (external treatment) and by absorption (internal treatment). Their effects are rapid, anything from a few minutes to up to four hours for physiological reactions.

Dermatoses

Racehorses often suffer from dermatoses (eczema, pruritus, alopecia, etc.). These are very common and may be of nervous origin or due to stress, or they may be the result of an unbalanced or over-rich diet, or even a reaction to allopathic medication. Here is a remarkable aromatic treatment: using a glove to avoid any irritation, apply hydrosol of cedar, followed by these mixtures (makes 1 litre of each):

Formula 1
oil of St John's wort	*600 ml*
EO of lavender or lavandin	*150 ml*
wheat germ oil	*250 ml*

Formula 2
oil of St John's wort	*100 ml*
wheat germ oil	*100 ml*
olive oil	*500 ml*
EO of rose geranium	*50 ml*
EO of rosemary	*50 ml*
EO of lavender	*150 ml*
EO of rose	*5 drops*
EO of sassafras	*50 ml*

Formula 3
*Comfort ABO**	*100 ml*
EO of lavender	*200 ml*
sesame oil	*600 ml*
wheat germ oil	*100 ml*

Alternate these three blends twice a day, taking care not to forget the preliminary gentle massage using hydrosol of cedar. Within a maximum of three days, the itching should stop.

* *ABO Confort from the Vie'Arôme laboratory, 13690 Graveson-en-Provence, France*

Comfort ABO for 100ml:

EO of rose geranium	*30ml*
EO of rose	*1ml*
Wheat germ oil	*30ml*
Sesame oil	*39ml*

Care and regrowth of the coat

After all attacks, knocks, bites, after-effects of dermatoses, wounds, and to keep the coat glossy and the mane in good condition, the following essential oils can be massaged in, using a circular movement, on the affected parts once or twice a day until the coat has completely recovered. Mix the essential oils with oil of St John's wort*, which is especially good as a decongestant and to promote formation of scar tissue.

* Note: Oil of St John's wort is obtained by macerating its flowers in cold-pressed virgin olive oil of less than 0.5 acidity, which ensures that it is excellent quality. Often a double maceration of flowers is carried out in the same oil. Its properties were made known at the beginning of the century by Dr Breuss (Germany), who also drew attention to its restorative qualities when he remarked that: "it reinflates intervertebral cartilage".

Essential oils for the care and regrowth of the coat
Formula 1

EO of cade	10 ml
EO of cedar	10 ml
EO of lavender	15 ml
EO of sage	10 ml
EO of thyme	5 ml
EO of ylang-ylang	10ml

to which you should add 60 ml of oil of St John's wort and 30 ml of wheat germ oil.

Formula 2

EO of terebinth	30 ml
EO of thyme	5 ml
EO of sage	10 ml
EO of ylang-ylang	15 ml

to which you should add 60 ml of oil of St John's wort and 30 ml of wheat germ oil.

This second formula should not be used before races, because of the presence of essential oil of terebinth.

For general maintenance, use 150 ml of either of the above mixtures in one litre of sesame oil. Formula 1 should be used after knocks, bites, or wounds that have closed in the first few days; then alternate formulas 1 and 2 until the coat has completely regrown. In certain cases, hydrosols of cedar, lavender and sage can be used initially to clean the wounds and prepare the skin for the effects of the essential oils. In stubborn cases, hydrosols can be used as an adjunct to other treatment.

To promote regrowth of a horse's tail
Use powdered ginger locally on the rectal area to encourage the animal to regrow the tail, a sign of vigour (Docteur Leclerc).

To summarise

We can appreciate just how important essential oils can be for our friend the horse - to promote health and happiness, to maintain general equilibrium, and to help acquire skills.

We should remember that all essential oils help to increase vitality and improve resistance to disease.

Just as for humans, the use of essential oils, albeit an excellent natural therapy, should never preclude consultation with the doctor or vet. The dosage and choice of appropriate essential oils, and their intelligent application, will give good results.

Often, results are rapid and long-lasting. If this is not the case, it would be advisable to consult your vet, some of whom are open to and competent in the practice of veterinary aromatherapy.

Before closing this chapter on the horse, I cannot resist the opportunity of letting you read several extracts from an ancient book, *l'Ecole de Cavalerie*, by Monsieur de la Guérinière of the Royal Stables, published in Paris in 1769.

l'Ecole de Cavalerie
by Monsieur de la Guérinière, Royal Stables

On the subject of sprains:

"If this first device does not cure the disease, then it is necessary to "pinch" the horse, that is to say, to bleed using an arterial clip, then to rub the fetlock joint with eau de vie and essence of terebinth, and then apply a poultice made from three half pints of urine, a quarter of olive oil and a peck of bran, having been twice brought to a rolling boil, placing poultice on a layer of oakum and applying warm to the area for treatment; leave for 24 hours, and repeat for five or six days. If the horse has improved, rub the area with eau de vie or balm of rosemary; if the horse has not improved, rub the affected part with a half pint of ardent balm and an equal amount of eau de vie.
Or here is another remedy: take bay oil, essence of terebinth and eau de vie; this is a type of blister remedy that the farriers call "dead fire", because it causes the coat to drop out ..."

On the subject of windgalls on the spavin or on the osselet of the fetlock ...

"After shaving the coat around the fetlock and on the windgall, apply the following ointment. Take two ounces each of cantharis (blister-flies), euphorbia and Christmas rose, grind to a powder, and make into an ointment with a sufficient quantity of equal amounts of oils of bay and of terebinth. Leave the ointment for some time ..."

On the subject of the inevitable injuries to the neck and withers ...

"(...) Use this only whilst waiting for the balm, for which

this is the recipe. Take six ounces of mineral oil, twelve ounces of essence of terebinth and a handful of hypericum* flowers, place together in a double glass bottle and leave in the sun for six weeks. Use as necessary."

* hypericum = St John's wort

Another remedy ...

"Take half an ounce each of Socotrine aloes and sugar, grind to a fine powder and mix with three ounces of oil of terebinth."

On the subject of purging, weight gain and stimulating the appetite ...

"Here is another technique that can be used. After having bled the horse, provided plain water and administered a purgative, you should feed it morning and evening with bran boiled in water, having previously mixed in on each occasion two ounces of the following powder, and half a peck of wheat.
Take two ounces each of: fenugreek, common salt, linseed, fennel seeds, anise seeds and bay seeds, sulphur flowers, liquorice, birthwort, agaric, myrrh, Socotrine aloes, and roots of the knapweed thistle, and one ounce each of clove, nutmeg, cinnamon and ginger. Grind to a fine powder prior to use".

On the subject of spirit and aromatic resolvents for sprains resulting from the horse falling down a precipice ...

"Take for example the lees of a good wine: bring to a boil and add a variety of herbs such as sage, thyme, rosemary, marjoram, bay, lavender, hyssop, etc. Cook well and mash, express juice through a strong, thick piece of linen or a press, and add to this: one quarter each of black pitch,

resin, and Burgundy pitch; two ounces of powdered Armeniac bole; one ounce each of bloodwort, mastic, frankincense and nut-gall; and two ounces each of oil of aspic (French lavender) and oil of terebinth. Boil together until the mixture has the consistency of a sticky, glue-like plaster, and then apply as hot as you are able without burning the animal, having previously rubbed all painful and affected parts with good quality eau de vie or spirit of wine. Then spread plaster over good quality fresh linen and suspend the horse for nine days".

On the subject of using a red plaster or a red honey-based ointment locally for sprains...

"Take two ounces each of cumin, fenugreek, bay berries and linseed; mix well together and add the following: eight ounces of wheatmeal, two ounces each of galbanum, bloodwort and mastic tears. Add to that eight ounces of essence of terebinth, Agrippa
ointment, and half a pound of thick pitch. Mix these thoroughly together ..."

On the subject of swelling of the thigh ...

"(...) and put appropriate honey-based ointment on the swollen part ... such as melted Montpellier ointment ... or make up a poultice using half a pound of thick pitch and an equal amount of common terebinth ... adding to that a quarter of bay oil."

On the subject of Montpellier ointment ...

As Montpellier ointment has been mentioned here, and as we have often recommended its use for the ailments covered in this book, we give here the recipe: it is very simple to make, since it only consists of mixing equal parts of poplar pommade (made from poplar buds, hog's fat and *solanaceous plants), althaea (marshmallow), and rose and honey ointment, mixed together cold in a vessel; this ointment is so effective that it can be used, if necessary, instead of a poultice or honey-based ointment.*

Take four ounces each of comfrey roots, pomegranate skin, bark of the oak tree, green cypress nuts and gall-nuts, seeds of the sumach and the barberry thorn-bush, two ounces each of aniseed and fennel seeds, two handfuls each of pomegranate flowers, camomile flowers and sweet clover flowers, and powdered crude alum ..."

On the subject of a Soleyfel plaster ...

"Take one ounce of galbanum, three ounces of ammoniacal gum and one and a half ounces of opopanax; leave mixture to infuse for two complete days in a pint pot of warm vinegar, then - and just as it is beginning to thicken - add four ounces each of black pitch and pitch resin and two ounces of terebinth. Mix together to make a plaster and apply to the affected part, renewing every nine days until the swelling has completely gone".

On the subject of swellings and injuries to the withers ...

"If it is a question of a simple suture on the withers without any abrasion, and if there is no reason to suspect internal bleeding, apply a liniment of bay oil, marshmallow ointment, and eau de vie, together with essence of terebinth and basil ..."

Those are just a few ancient remedies for horses in which essence of terebinth, bay oil, essence of lavender or of aspic (French lavender) are common. The red-coloured oil made with the flowers of St John's wort (hypericum) was also in common use.

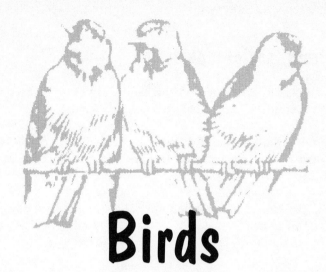

Birds

Canaries, parrots, mynah birds

Suffering, as they do, from a lack of freedom, caged birds are delicate. In addition to the usual diet and care you give them, the provision of an essential oil treatment by diffusion will help in the following cases:

Respiratory problems

The bird's most important function is its breathing: you could describe it as a "flying lung".

For respiratory problems, use an electric aromatic diffuser, several times a day, near the cage, for periods of 5 minutes each.

Respiratory essential oil blend for the diffuser
EO of eucalyptus	10 ml
EO of pine	5 ml
EO of tea-tree	2 ml
EO of niaouli or cajeput	3 ml

Stress, anxiety, dejection

Essential oils for these problems can be used in a diffuser or taken internally:

- for internal treatment: 1 drop of essential oil of neroli for mynah birds, ¼ drop for parrots and canaries, twice a day, for 3 to 7 days.

- for diffusion: 5 minutes near the cage 4 to 5 times a day:

EO of lavender	*10 ml*
EO of marjoram	*4 ml*
EO of neroli	*1 ml*

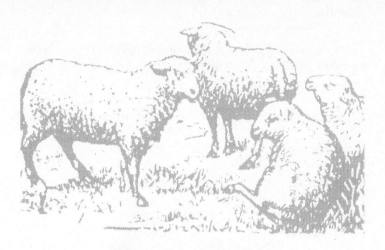

Rearing

Calves, cows, pigs, goats, sheep ...

Placing the aromatic diffuser in the animal house is the simplest method of using essential oils in caring for livestock, at least in the treatment of infectious and respiratory diseases.

The diffuser can be left on indefinitely at the rate of 2 to 5 ml an hour, 2 hours a day as a prophylactic, and 12 to 24 hours a day as a curative treatment.

Essential oils can also be added to food (5 to 10 drops a day of the selected essential oil or oils).

Revitalising treatments can be carried out 2 to 3 times a year as a preventative measure. Don't forget that all essential oils are antiseptic, increase resistance to disease, promote elimination of toxins and parasites, and revitalise by giving new energy.

Respiratory blend for the diffuser or for internal use (makes 1 litre)

EO of eucalyptus	450 ml
EO of pine	150 ml
EO of thyme	50 ml
EO of rosemary	50 ml
EO of terebinth	200 ml
EO of tea-tree	100 ml

Anti-infectious blend for diffuser or ingestion (makes 1 litre)

EO of thyme	100 ml
EO of wild marjoram	150 ml
EO of lavandin	300 ml
EO of rosemary	300 ml
EO of cinnamon (bark)	50 ml
EO of basil	100 ml

For specific infections, consult the *Table of principal ailments* and/or the chapter on *Horses*.

The normal dose for a 50 kg animal is 5 drops, twice a day, in food for 3 weeks as a preventative measure, or one week in acute cases.

In the diffuser the blend can be used regularly.

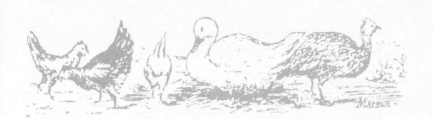

Rearing

Chickens, hens, ducks, geese ...

When it comes to rearing our two-footed friends, respiratory problems and minor infections are dealt with by using an aromatic diffuser containing an appropriate blend of essential oils.

The size of the bird house will determine the length of use, depending on the model used.

For an area of 50 sq m, you will need to diffuse approximately 2 ml per hour for 3 to 12 hours a day for 2 to 3 days, and then, for maintenance, 1 to 2 hours per day for 10 days.

Respiratory blend for the diffuser (makes 1 litre)
EO of eucalyptus	*450 ml*
EO of pine	*150 ml*
EO of thyme	*50 ml*
EO of rosemary	*50 ml*
EO of terebinth	*200 ml*
EO of tea-tree	*100 ml*

Anti-infectious aromatic blend (makes 1 litre)

EO of thyme	*100 ml*
EO of wild marjoram	*150 ml*
EO of lavandin	*300 ml*
EO of rosemary	*300 ml*
EO of cinnamon (bark)	*50 ml*
EO of basil	*100 ml*

For specific ailments, 1 to 3 drops per day in food brings rapid improvement. Hydrosols can also be used: refer to the *Table of principal ailments* at the beginning of this book.

Tactics for
warding off pests

Flies

Place some whole cloves, which have been boiled, on a plate. Rehumidify as necessary. Or insert cloves into an orange and add a few drops of essential oil of cloves.

Mosquitoes and small biting insects, harvest mites and spiders

Citronella is effective in diffusion against mosquitoes; however, unfortunately, its odour strangely resembles the products available for cleaning toilets. A mixture without citronella but dominated by cinnamon and 27 other essential oils* has proved to be especially effective. It is an anti-inflammatory product, and soothes the pain of bites from spiders, mosquitoes, ants and all flying insects.

Cats

Essential oil of exotic verbena repels cats.

* Stop'moustic (anti mosquito product) - laboratoire vie'Arôme - 13690 Graveson-en-Provence, France.

Index of ailments

Birds

anxiety, 92
dejection, 92
respiratory problems, 91
stress, 92

Cats

abraded pads, 28
abscesses, 27
anaemia, 24
anorexia, 24
coryza, 31
coughs, 30
emphysema, 30
exhaustion, 23
fatigue, 23
feeding, 21
fleas, 29
fractures, 32
giving birth, 22
intestinal parasites, 26
odours, 33
paws, 28
poisoning, 25
thorns/splinters/spikelets, 28
typhus, 31
weight loss, 24
worming, 26

Dogs

abraded pads, 55
abscesses, 54
anaemia, 50
anorexia, 50
bacterial infections, 53
breath, 64
coat, 15, 63
dermatoses, 60, 62
exhaustion, 48
fatigue, 49
feeding, 38–40, 42, 43–4
fleas, 62
fractures, 56
giving birth, 41
infectious diseases, 53
paralysis, 57, 59
paws, 55
poisoning, 51
pregnancy, 40
puppies, 43–4
purgatives, 52
rheumatism, 57–8
skin diseases, 60
small shot, 61
suckling, 42
thorns/spinters/spikelets, 55
ticks, 61
vaccinations, 45
weight loss, 50
worming, 46–7

Bibliography

Pharmacopée universelle, Emery (d'), édition d'Haury, 1697.

Manuel de l'Ecole de Cavalerie, Monsieur de la Guérinière, Ecuyer du Roi, published in Paris by La Compagnie, 1769.

Perfumes and essential oils, Holmes, Record, 1912-1913.

Aromathérapie and *Antiseptiques essentiels*, R.M. Gattefossé, Girardot, 1923 republished in English by The C.W. Daniel Company, Saffron Walden, England; librairie des Sciences, 1957.

Travaux aromathérapie vétérinaire, Docteur Louis Sévelinge, published by the author, Bourg-de-Thizy.

The Practice of Aromatherapy Docteur Jean Valnet, The C.W. Daniel Company, Saffron Walden, England, 1977.

Dictionnaire médical du chien, Stephen Schneck and Dr Nigel Norris, éditions Marabout, 1981.

Le Guide santé de votre chien, Professeur J.P. Cottet and Docteur H. Laforge, éditions Atlas, 1986.

Dictionnaire des médecines douces pour chiens et chats, Luce Bonnefous et Docteur Peker, éditions du Rocher, 1986.

How to prescribe herbal medicines, the Mediherb Prescriber Reference, compiled by K. Bone, N. Burgess, D. McLeod. Mediherb, 1992.

The Journal of Essential Oil Research, vol. 4, number 4, July-August 1992, published by Allured Publishing Corporation, USA.

Aromathérapie, santé et bien-être par les huiles essentielles éditions Albin Michel, 1993 and *Aromathérapie 2, des huiles essentielles pour votre santé*, Nelly Grosjean, éditions de la chevêche, 1991.

Aromatherapy from Provence, Nelly Grosjean, The C.W. Daniel Company, Saffron Walden, England, 1993.

Useful addresses and information

Some French veterinary aromatherapy specialists

Laboratoire Aromathérapie Vie'Arôme
la chevêche, 13690 Graveson-en-Provence, France
Natural and "organic" quality aromatic essential oils, hydrosols, aromatic diffusers, books on aromatherapy and Nelly Grosjean's aromatic specialities. Mail order facility. Delivery within 48 hours in France, 5 days elsewhere.
Tel (+ 33) 90 95 81 72 Fax (+ 33) 90 95 85 20.

Laboratoire Diétaroma
BP 4 - 69240 Bourg-de-Thizy, France
Products based on essential oils and natural plant extracts. Products available from health food shops and chemists.
Fax (+33) 74 64 17 25

Laboratoire Néo-Lupus
BP 49 - 33313 Arcachon Cedex, France
Founded in 1934, Néo-lupus and Azymic specialist natural products based on aromatic plants. Available from chemists.

"Natural" livery for horses
Haras du Jaunay - Ste Hélène
85220 L'Aiguillon-sur-Vie, France
Tel (+ 33) 51 22 83 42 or (+ 33) 47 09 02 32 (Paris)
Equine breeding, livery, convalescence. Showpiece of natural medicine for horses (organically grown fodder, oligotherapy, nutritherapy). Dr Jacques Leguern, natural therapy vet and consultant for those living outside France.

Information on natural veterinary medicine

IMEV (training and communications organisation, director
Docteur Alain Bouchet, veterinarian)
2 rue du Vieux Bassin
30700 Montaren, France
Tel (+ 33) 66 22 57 55 Fax (+ 33) 66 22 45 98

• Professional Training
Veterinary and comparative osteopathy (for medical
profession only), veterinary acupuncture (for vets only),
geobiology.

• Courses, seminars, organised trips
Geobiology, cosmography and associated therapies, medical
divination (radiation detection), natural therapies, personal
development.

• Veterinary meetings (subscription available)
Quarterly journal devoted to natural animal therapies.

LA CHEVECHE ASSOCIATION
Petite route du grès 13690 Graveson-en-Provence, France.

• TRAINING COURSES IN AROMATHERAPY by Nelly Grosjean
(France, Switzerland, United States, Asia)
On demand, for groups of 15 people or more.
Special course available for doctors, therapists and vets.
Information on all courses on (+ 33) 90 95 81 55 Fax (+33) 90
95 85 20.

Vie'Arome

Nelly Grosjean's natural products
la chevêche - 13690 Graveson-en-Provence, France
Tel (+ 33) 90 95 81 72 Fax (+ 33) 90 95 85 20

Mail order sales.

Aromatic diffusers

To breathe is to live. It is the primary function of the body. "We can stop drinking or eating for a few days, but we can't stop breathing for more than a few minutes." Electrically powered, the aromatic diffuser disperses into the air billions of micro particles of essential oils, without heating them, through an ingenious system of cold air vaporisation, consisting of a pump and a clear pyrex container. You can use this aromatic diffuser and associated essential oils to create a fragrant atmosphere in your house which will be effective in protecting your home against microbes and various forms of pollution. The diffuser regenerates, cleanses, ionises, enriches, revitalises and perfumes the air that you breathe. Many models available for both home and professional use.

Mixtures for aromatic diffusers

Exotic verbena is the essential oil of happiness and communication! All essential oils modify and improve the olfactory ambience of home, office, waiting room and public places.

• SEDATIVES: *lavender-lavandin, orange, relaxant, harmony, bio-relax*

• TONICS: *tonic, freshtonic, bio-fresh, hammam, lemon*

• AMBIANCE: *anti-tobacco, Christmas ambiance, summer garden, exotic verbena, anti-mosquito.*

• RESPIRATORY: *eucalyptus, bio-respir, tonic, forest.*

• "BIO": *superior lavender from Provence, eucalyptus, bio-respir, bio-fresh, bio-relax, pine, lavandin, terebinth.*

My twelve essential oil massages

Perfumed oil was originally used in Egypt as a balm or ointment made from flowers or plants prepared by the priest, doctor or oracle, for the health of the body and spirit. It can be used in the morning or evening to promote physical and mental well-being, loving qualities, confidence, creativity or communication. Just as there are twelve moons, twelve months, twelve signs of the zodiac and twelve apostles, so my twelve massage preparations can be used to address twelve common problems of daily life.

Developed over more than fifteen years, they correspond to the twelve metabolic functions of our remarkable human body. An essential oil massage preparation harmonises, balances, tones, relaxes and soothes; as the perfume envelops the flower, so these essential oils protect us from the rigours of daily life and bring our body vital, renewed energy.

With their properties of protection, harmony, vitality and regeneration, my twelve massage preparations both store and restore nature's vital elements, bringing us extra energy essential for our well-being. You will enjoy the benefits of them both morning and evening, and soon you won't be able to do without them!

APH ACTION:	*Alertness, equilibrium, sexual drive, vitality*
NER RELAX:	*Inner peace, promotes sleep*
HAR HARMONY:	*Relaxation, meditation, yoga*
RES RESPIRATORY:	*Purification and natural immunity*
RHU PAIN RELIEF:	*Soothes pain*
CEL:	*Toning up veins, soft tissue filtration*

VIT VITALITY: *Success in exams and competitions, increased drive and dynamism*

DIG DIGESTION: *Good digestion*

MIN SLIMMING: *Detoxification of the body, weight control*

106 HAIR: *Promotes beautiful hair, stimulates hair follicle*

107 MASTERPIECE: *Tissue regenerator, anti-ageing remedy*

109 LEGS/FEET: *Promotes good circulation, renews and refreshes*

IN THE U.S.A.
Vie Arôme's products are distributed by;
Aromatherapy International,
3 Seal Harbor Road, Suite 437,
Winthrop, MA 02152
tel: 617 846 0285 fax: 617 846 5474

Aromatic body oils
(for the bath, body, face and around the eyes)

The six aromatic body oils consist of oils from cereal grains, fruits or herbs in synergy with aromatic essential oils (35 to 40%). These are natural products and contain no preservatives or synthetic chemicals. Rich in noble vitamins, their active aromatic properties make these oils remarkable for their regenerative, anti-ageing and revitalising qualities. ABO TONIC, ABO RELAX, ABO FRESH, ABO COMFORT, ABO FACE, ABO EYES.

Hydrosols

Vie'Arôme hydrosols are produced from the first 20 litres of water from each distillation of aromatic plants, untreated and organically grown on our land at Sault, and distilled with spring water.
A slight sediment may form on the surface after a few months, in which case filtering will be all that is required.

HOW DO I USE THEM?

- as a daily drink
- as a "sugarfree" syrup
- on the hair
- for smarting skin after shaving
- for veterinary purposes
- as a rapid infusion
- in the bath
- for the eyes
- for the face

Fragrances to create a particular ambience

These vapourisers, very practical for the house, the car or the boat, are available as a 50 ml or 100 ml spray: *freshtonic, orange-mandarin, exotic verbena, relaxant, oriental with cinnamon, respiratory.*

Massage oils 125 ml

DES mystic (myrrh, myrtle, sandalwood, hyssop)
LOU trekking (geranium, rosemary, camomile, rose)

Anti-mosquito

Spray 15 ml
Repels mosquitoes, soothes all bites and stings.

Full details of Vie Arôme products may be obtained by writing to;
  Laboratoire Aromathérapie Vie 'Arome la chevêche,
  13690 Graveson-en-Provence, France
and asking for a copy of 'the little catalogue'.

Visit the museum of fragrances and perfume in Graveson-en- Provence

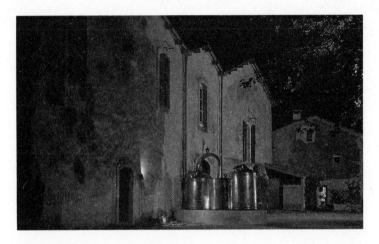

From fragrances to perfumes ...

Located in the heart of Provence between Alpilles and Montagnette, near les Baux, Fontvielle and the mill of Daudet, near Maillane, the homeland of Frédéric Mistral, and Tarascon, dominated by the famous Tartarin castle, the museum promises you a heady, exciting journey. Cypress hedges protect the experimental garden where varieties of lavender and lavandin, savory, sage, camomile, mint, verbena, wild marjoram, sweet marjoram, cornflower, inula, St John's wort and milfoil are grown organically, a paradise of new fragrances and colours for foreign visitors discovering the thousand and one delights of Provence.

La chevêche, petite route du grès,
13690 Graveson-en-Provence, France
Tel 90 95 81 55 Fax 90 95 85 20

Index

for dermatoses, 81
for exhaustion, 48
for fatigue, 49
for fur loss, 16
for joint pains, 77, 78
for muscular pains, 76
for respiratory problems, 74,
  94, 95, 96
for rheumatism, 57
for scar tissue healing, 16
in tonic for horses, 69
rosewood
for circulation, 79
for skin diseases, 60
for skin problems, 80

S

sage
for circulation, 79
for coat, 83
for giving birth, 22, 41
St John's wort, 15, 79, 83
for abscesses, 54, 72
for circulation, 79
for coat, 83
for cutaneous lesions, 16
for cuts, 16
for dermatoses, 81
for fur loss, 16
for joint pains, 77
for muscular pains, 76
for relaxation, 16
for rheumatism, 57
for scar tissue healing, 16
for skin diseases, 60
for skin problems, 80
for sores, 16
for thorns, 28, 55
for ticks, 61
sandalwood, 2
sassafras
for dermatoses, 81
in vermifuge, 26
for worming, 46, 73
savory, 5
for bacterial/infectious
  diseases, 53
for coryza, 31
for typhus, 31
scar formation promotion *see*
  cicatrisants
scar tissue healing, 16
scratches, 11

sedative oils, 14, 15, 104
sheep, 93–4
skin problems, 8
  dogs, 60
  horses, 80
sleep inducers, 14
slimming oils, 14
small shot, dogs, 61
smell, of oils, 2
snake bite, 11
Soleyfel plaster, 89
sores, 11
spicules *see* thorns
spiders, 97
spikelets *see* thorns
splinters *see* thorns
sprains, 11
  horses, 86, 87–8
staphylococci, 11
stiffness, horses, 77–8
stings, 11
Stop'moustic, 97
streptococci *see* staphylococci
stress
  birds, 92
  horses, 70–1
  and see distress
suckling, dogs, 42
sweet marjoram
  for joint pains, 77
  for stress, 70, 71
sweet thyme, for joint pains, 78
swellings, horses, 88, 89 *and see*
  inflammation

T

tartar, 11
taste, of oils, 2
tea-tree, for respiratory
problems, 30, 74, 91, 94, 95
tendon inflammation, horses, 76
  and see inflammation
terebinth, 15
for coat, 63, 83
for cuts, 16
for fleas, 62
for joint pains, 77, 78
for muscular pains, 76
for odours, 33
for respiratory problems, 74,
  94, 95
for rheumatism, 57
for skin diseases, 60